I0758845

The Power of Extracise

Increase Your Body Awareness

Christian Karl

Edition 1.2

Copyright© 2023 by author Christian Karl. All Rights Reserved. Registered with the U.S. Copyright Office.

I dedicate this book to all those who have a burning interest in getting deeper into the mystery of existence.

Table Of Contents

Table Of Contents 4

Preface 7

About The Author 9

Why Did I Write This Book? 11

Introduction 13

Getting Deeper Into It 15

The Extracise Mission.............................. 17

Motivation... 18

Thoughts On Competitiveness................. 21

Purpose And Intent 23

A Story About Two Hindu Sages 27

Form Follows Function............................ 28

The Deeper Practice................................ 30

My Personal Experience Practicing Extracise........ 33

Take A Body Inventory 35

Where To Practice.................................... 36

The Need for A Purpose 37

Personal Experiences.............................. 39

On The Practice 42

My Spiritual Path................................... 45

On Pain 46

My Mornings and Evenings.................... 49

The Phases Of The Breath................................... 50

The Final Breath 51

The State Of Magnificence.............................. 55

Awareness.. 56

Meditate On Bliss.. 57

The Body Speaks To You 58

Personal Experiences.................................... 61

Paying Attention 62

A Breathing Practice...................................... 64

Where To Focus During The Practice.................... 66

Thoughts On Walking, Jogging, and Running 69

Mobility And Flexibility 70

About The Workout 72

Use Of A Mantra 75

About Reversal Of The Fluids............................ 76

General Guidelines On Positions 79

Your Personal Practice 80

Thoughts On Using Weights And TRX Straps........ 82

A Personal experience 83

On The Health Industry.................................... 85

Thoughts On Inner Functions Vs. Outer Forms 87

Some Basic Extracise Starting Positions 89

A Sample Extracise Session 93

Thoughts On The Practice................................. 96

More On Pain 98

The Conscious Will 100

On Perfection 101

About Food And Drinks 102

Extracise Highlights 103

Deep Belly Breathing............................. 105

Follow The Breath 106

Thoughts On Holding Poses 107

Before Bedtime 108

Loading Of The Bones 109

This Body... 110

Flow of Chi... 111

Human Efforts Towards Higher Aspiration 112

Primer On The Assemblage Point 114

Final Thoughts..................................... 117

And ... The Wrap-up 123

Other Books By The Author 125

Contact Information............................... 125

Preface

Too many people are dependent on painkillers. The first line of defense of the body's health is a regular and consistent exercise routine. This book offers such a routine that is simple, easy, and will leave you feeling great within your skin.

It is important to get the body ready for the eventuality of a stumble, a trip-up, a push or a shove, a more serious accident, an operation, the breaking of a bone, the twisting of an ankle, the pulling of a muscle, and so on. It is prudent to have a body that is ready to deal with these challenges in the best possible way by being flexible and adaptable.

When a muscle or a tendon does not get used a lot, then it cannot respond properly to sudden challenges that might arise. What if you tripped and caught yourself, but pulled a muscle in the process? If that muscle is flexible and strong, then you might only suffer some minor discomfort for a short time. But if you hadn't used that muscle in a while, then pulling it might cause you great discomfort and may keep you out of circulation a lot longer.

My two strong motivations to exercise are: keeping the body working properly and keeping any discomfort to a minimum. I found that when I keep up my routine consistently, then I feel physically and mentally great, since my body is in good condition and my mind is free to enjoy the day.

Many people who suffer chronic physical pain also feel mentally and emotionally drained. They exhaust more easily and are disinclined to participate in fun activities, which puts a damper on their quality of life.

About The Author

I am a dedicated practitioner of Yoga, Meditation, Self-inquiry, Chi Kung, and Isometric energizing techniques. With over fifty years of experience, these practices have become an integral part of my daily life.

My dedication to these techniques stems from my desire to increase sensitivity and deepen awareness. Through consistent practice, I have discovered the transformative power of these modalities and the profound impact they can have on one's physical, mental, and emotional well-being.

My approach to these practices is rooted in mindfulness and self-awareness. I believe that by being present and fully engaged in the moment, we can tap into a deeper level of consciousness and unlock our full potential. This philosophy has helped me to develop a sense of inner peace and calm, even in the midst of life's challenges.

I am constantly exploring new techniques and modalities, seeking to deepen my understanding and enhance my practice. I am passionate about sharing my knowledge and experiences with others and I am always eager to learn from fellow practitioners.

Why Did I Write This Book?

I wanted to share my love of Extracise, the bliss I've experienced and continue to experience doing it.

There is a deep sense of gratitude and appreciation in my heart and mind for being able to practice it. I love my body and mind for assisting me on this marvelous journey of life.

This book is a collection of notes, journal entries, and frequent contemplations over the years on a subject that is so very dear to my heart: my body and its harmonious functioning.

So, what is Extracise? It is a system of individualized body movements combined with the conscious will that I developed utilizing many of the various exercise regimens I have encountered thus far.

I use the term "Extracise", because extracise is defined as "The act of engaging in extra exercise, beyond one's normal regimen." It is that extra effort we exert, that extra conscious will we employ to get deeper into the breath, deeper into the stretch, deeper into the muscle contraction, deeper into the muscle relaxation, deeper into all of the aspects of this extraordinary body of ours to gain a deeper understanding of it through our practice.

Right now, what "extra" can you do right now while reading these words that you'd normally not be doing? You could, for example, consciously wiggle your little finger and become aware of its muscles. That would be something extra. You could consciously sit up and stretch your spine to feel the energy flow more freely.

In every one of your life's situations, whatever they are, you can always add something extra. When sitting, what can you add? When running, you could pay extra attention to your physical activity and your breathing, and go deeper into your body awareness. When practicing yoga, you could consciously breathe deeper into the poses and free yourself thereby from ingrained impurities. The same with Chi Kung and other modalities.

One of the concepts I hold dear comes from architecture and it is this: "Form follows Function." That is how I approach my workouts. First, I listen to the inner needs of my body and then I exercise my joints, muscles, and tendons in such a way as to answer those needs; always with my awareness focused on finding the deepest sense of inner harmony and the most blissful experience of being.

Introduction

I gained my first experience with truly beneficial physical exercises when I was about twenty years old, so this is ancient history, now that I am sixty-nine.

When I got drafted into the army, after being denied conscientious objector status, the examining physician placed a measuring tape along the lower area of my spine, had me bend forward, and immediately told me: "you are out of here!" I was astonished to hear that, because I had no idea that I had such a severe back problem. I had been experiencing constant burning down into my legs, but that had been going on for as long as could remember, and it had become part of my existence. Yes, it was uncomfortable and at times debilitatingly painful, but since it was constant, I had gotten used to it.

Now that I had learned that there was something seriously wrong with my spine, I went to see two doctors. The first told me he could fix a loose connection between two vertebrae by fusing them together. That solution did not get me excited. Then I saw a second doctor, which I believe was a chiropractor. He recommended an easy set of isometric back muscle strengthening exercises to take some of the weight off the spine. This sounded better to me, so I tried his approach.

Lying on my bed with the arms on my sides, I simply pressed down with my left leg and my right arm for a few seconds. Then I repeated that with the other leg and arm. I also pressed down with both legs and arms simultaneously. So simple!

After a few days of practice, to my great surprise, the burning sensation down into my legs disappeared! All of a sudden, I was pain-free! I felt liberated! What a relief! I couldn't believe that this easy daily workout had done the trick.

I realized how debilitating this burning sensation had been all along, and I continued to practice the prescribed therapy. I am not saying that it fixed the underlying cause, which was a loose connection between two vertebrae, but that it helped me manage the condition I was born with. I have continued strengthening my back and stomach muscles and have been able to keep the condition under control.

Getting Deeper Into It

After I experienced this profound impact on my sense of wellbeing, I tried various body, mind, and breath workouts and developed a fondness for experiences that connected me with deeper and deeper levels within myself. The deeper I got, the more pleasant were the sensations I found, until I came to the source of it all, the blissful underlying state of being. Here I found that my conscious will, and my listening awareness merged in a unity of feeling great, of feeling alive – of feeling a deep sense of blissful existence.

I began listening more and more within my body and looked for inner ways of dealing with any sensation of discomfort. As a next step, I shifted the focus from alleviating discomforts to feeling good, better, and even great within my skin.

I practiced Yoga, Chi Kung, and Isometrics and over time realized that my focus always needed to be "inner" directed – finding ways through awareness and through listening to the body of vitalizing all parts of the body, joints, muscles, and tendons, not neglecting even the smallest ones, such as the eyelids. In other words, I needed to give extra attention to it all.

And let's not forget the brain, the most important organ of the body. How to stimulate it? Breathe consciously into it. Draw the breath in through your spine and breathe into an imaginary brain center. Send your attention and breath upwards to the brain and feel it get vitalized.

The Extracise Mission

The mission of Extracise is to use the conscious will to fully bend or rotate every joint, fully contract and relax every muscle, fully stretch every muscle and tendon — while breathing with the clearest awareness into and out of the joints, the muscles, and the tendons. And doing all this while paying the closest attention of the effects of these exercises on your body and mind!

All the components of your body are necessary. They are all here to serve a purpose, and they all deserve our closest attention. They should all act together in harmony when we exercise them and create a sense of wellbeing that makes us feel invigorated, comfortable and balanced. And ultimately supremely blissful!

Motivation

Why would you want to Extracise? A good motivation would be to explore your own body more fully – that extraordinary vehicle carrying you so faithfully through life. It is the only tool you have to work with in your existence. You might as well become familiar with it. Learn its strengths and weaknesses. And then take it for a spin!

Extracise is, like everything else in life, a tool for self-discovery.

First of all, you need to know what lies behind the skin that covers you from head to toe. There are muscles, tendons, nerves, ligaments, blood vessels, and trillions of cells forming all kinds of necessary organs.

Your conscious will can influence just about all these components of your body. That is what the practice of Extracise is all about.

You may be curious about what is going on inside your body, and your awareness can tell you all about it. You can sense when you are uptight, when your blood pressure is too high, when you are unbalanced, when you are out of shape, when your energy level is down.

You can use your conscious effort to get yourself uplifted and energized, make yourself feel better, strengthened, and comfortable. You do not need to focus on specific external forms; all you need to do is focus on your internal needs and then let your efforts flow from there.

Extracise encompasses the entire range of moving, as well as still physical forms, based on your personal inner needs.

An easy way to begin an Extracise practice is to consciously breathe in and out several times while being fully aware of the energy flow into and through your body. Focus deeply! Keep the stomach muscles relaxed! Sense the tingling vibrations invigorate you from your brain to your toes.

After this, you can add the following simple practice: while sitting or standing comfortably, use your conscious will to gently contract the biceps of your right arm in three steps on the in-breaths: from relaxed to mild to medium to max. Hold the contraction for a few seconds together with your breath, and then breathe out and release the muscles in the same three steps from max to medium to mild, and then to complete relaxation.

Then practice with the left arm. Be fully aware. Use your inner, conscious will alone to perform this Extracise. Remove your ego completely. There is no doer; there is only Doing!

To fully exercise your body in this way, repeat this with all the muscles of your body that you have access to. Use your conscious will in an extra concentrated way to get the most out of this practice. The more focused you are, the more you'll get to know your body and the more you'll experience its magnificence.

Thoughts On Competitiveness

We humans have become very competitive over the years. Unfortunately, this exaggerated competitive drive has infiltrated the health and fitness regimes of people.

Higher, faster, better, more, etc., have become the yardsticks for success in sports and fitness.

That is not the way to finding a sense of true inner balance in your body and mind. You cannot be constantly striving for something external while simultaneously searching for inner harmony and a sense of balanced wellbeing in your physical workouts.

These externally directed and goal-oriented efforts will not lead to peace of mind. They may result in a – often times short-lived – sense of accomplishment and pride once you have been given that acknowledgment of your achievement.

Permanent inner peace and harmony cannot arise from a "must achieve" chase after something that is dangling in front of your vision, but that will ultimately always be just one step ahead of you.

There is also a tendency to measure everything scientifically, to categorize it, to compare numbers, to enter it into a value system, to organize things from 1st to last place. "And the winner is…!" We are forgetting that when there are winners, there are also losers. Who wants to be in last place? Based on this system, there will always be more losers than winners. How does this contribute to peace of mind and a sense of harmony in your life?

Purpose And Intent

Always engage in your Extracise practice with a clear sense of purpose and willful direction. Never automatic, never without paying extra close attention. That is why I like to shut my eyes so I can go deeply into the practice.

You can practice outdoors or indoors, morning, noon, or night. It doesn't matter when or where. It is only important that you do it. Comfortable and safe spaces with plenty of fresh air would be best.

Sample session: Stand with your feet a bit apart, arms at your sides, face towards the sun or an open window, and keep the eyes closed. Practice barefoot on a mat, or wear non-slip socks, or comfortable shoes. Don't let your feet get cold.

Now explore your body like a toddler would, who has just learned to stand on their own two feet. Move your limbs this way and that. Stretch. Reach. Bend. Contract. Relax. Twist. Wiggle.

Really focus on what you are doing. Be aware of every nuance of your movements, muscle activity, sense of balance, sense of flowing motion, sense of contracting and relaxing of muscles. Awareness is paramount. It is the key.

If you are outside, let the sun's rays penetrate you. "Namaste to the Sun," greetings to the sun, welcoming its warmth, vitality, and energy. Feel great inside your skin.

As a suggestion, you may want to start your body exploration with your toes, and then move on to your feet, your calves, your thighs, your buttocks, your hip, your lower back, your upper back, your lower stomach, your upper stomach, your chest, your back, your shoulders, your fingers, hands, and lower arms, your upper arms, front and back of your neck, your entire face with all its parts, your scalp.

Always breathe deeply and with full awareness into any joint movement and muscle contraction. This will help guide your mind to these areas, which will tell you exactly what is going on there and make you aware of any problems you need to deal with in the moment.

Don't strain. Take it easy. At first you may not be able to locate and activate some of your muscles, but over time, with practice and patience, you will get access to most of them.

Your all-important heart muscle can be worked on indirectly, as I am explaining later on.

Fully relax the joints, muscles, and tendons after using them, especially after holding a body position for a while. In this relaxed state your mind will tell you much about the status of your joints, muscles, and tendons. Only begin another position after you have learned everything there is to know about the present one.

In a way, you are very much embracing each position by understanding exactly what your body is getting from it.

The focus of Extracise is the awareness of your body and its inner energies right here, right now. Allow this energy to pull you in and see what you find there: vitality – bliss – peace – love – freedom.

Have reverence for this moment and gratitude for being here, for being alive, to be able to experience this life with your senses, mind, and spirit. Find you true home in the sizzling world of inner consciousness.

The external body forms you are using during Extracise are a reflection of the needs of your body's joints, muscles, and tendons while you are attempting to find comfort and ease inside.

Only you know what kind of workout your body needs in this moment: fast or slow, holding a pose or changing it, remaining still or swaying side to side, bending forwards or backwards, etc.

Perhaps you want to rock gently back and forth while breathing in and out of the focal point in your head where all sensory impressions merge.

You know when it is time to begin an exercise and when it is time to stop. Only you know what particular forms your body needs to feel in the perfect zone of invigorated harmony and blissful balance. This could be a still form or a moving form.

A still form is a body position where you don't move any joints. You are breathing into muscles while you are consciously contracting them.

A moving form is a body position or form, where you are moving joints. You are breathing into these moving joints. You are also breathing into contracting muscles. These moving forms can be stationary, as when you perform them on a mat, or moving, as in running on a treadmill, or rowing a boat. The choice is always yours. Whatever makes you happy! There are no restrictions on your movements. But you always need to keep the focus as much as possible within yourself to get the most benefit from your exercise.

The goal of Extracise is always the same: use your conscious will to fully bend or rotate every joint, fully flex every muscle, fully stretch every muscle and tendon. Consciously breathe into and out of your joints, muscles, and tendons. Be aware of your efforts on your body and mind.

A Story About Two Hindu Sages

I read a story about two sages in a Hindu scripture. One sage said that in order to get the full benefit of a Mantra, one had to repeat it 100,000 times. The other sage said that if you were to repeat the Mantra with the full awareness of its essence, then you would only need to repeat it once.

The latter is how I feel about workouts, and that's why I developed my system of Extracise. One deeply conscious performance of an exercise with the full awareness of its effect on the body and mind is often enough to make you feel great. Multiple repetitions are no guarantee to increase this level of wellbeing.

Form Follows Function

I am great believer in the dictum that "Form follows Function." In the context of this exercise system, it means that the outer Form your body assumes follows from the inner Function that your awareness leads you to.

I observe that many people chase the outer Form in order to find the inner Function of wellbeing. It is true to some extent that if you follow a pre-prescribed Form, you will reap certain health rewards. Established forms also provide some cover for criticism. Following your own inner directives can be scary, especially if you feel you are being judged. This judge can be yourself. Self-censuring is a habit that is deeply ingrained in many of us.

"Trust but verify." That is great advice. Practice whatever workout someone suggests, and then see for yourself what it does to your sense of wellbeing. Only you are the judge of that. That's when it truly becomes valuable to you. And that's when you want to add it to your workout repertoire. "Take the honey." Take the essence and enjoy it.

The most inner experience you'll ever have is the notion of "I am alive, I exist." Extracise can make you feel deeply alive in this precious moment with the assistance of the conscious will that you use to activate all your body parts, from head to toe.

The forms you choose during your practice are solely based on your inner needs.

Every Extracise practice is a "right" Extracise practice, if done with your full awareness observing its effects, while breathing consciously and fully into your activities, using your will energy. Go deeper and deeper into your poses, into your body positions.

A certain degree of elegance develops after practicing for a while. This elegance is the result of economy of form gracefully done. Done to perfection!

The Deeper Practice

Extracise is an intentional practice, where you use your conscious will to accomplish something inside your body, inside the barrier of the skin that covers your body from head to toe. You cannot always see what you are doing, but you can feel it, you can sense the results. You feel the air stream into your lungs, then sense it invigorating your body, then comes the necessary exhale, followed by more invigorating intakes of vital oxygen and energy. And so on.

Using your conscious mind, locate and contract various muscles or muscle groups. This will increase the blood flow into the muscles, the tendons, and whatever else surrounds them. You can practice this to revitalize your muscles and energize various body parts.

You do not have to move your body to practice Extracise. You can appear to be sitting, standing, or lying perfectly still, but underneath your skin you are actively involved in stimulating your muscles and thereby invigorating your body.

It is relatively easy to direct your attention to any part of your body by taking a conscious breath, and then directing the energy flow by breathing into any muscle while contracting it.

Your will directs your conscious efforts. The clearer your intention is, the more concentrated, the quicker you will feel the results of your efforts.

Concentrated, directed, conscious will is the key to Extracise.

Every contraction of your muscles has an effect on your heart, because muscles act like pumps when contracting and relaxing. They act either in concert with the heart pump or against it. In the first instance they release the pressure on the heart, thereby lowering your blood pressure. In the second instance, they increase the pressure on your heart, thereby increasing your blood pressure.

Whenever you are contracting muscles while the heart is pumping blood, then you are adding to the resistance of your body to the blood flow and are forcing your heart muscle to work a bit harder, thereby exercising your heart muscle.

The important aspect to remember when it comes to Extracise is that you are using your conscious will to affect your muscles, nerves, tendons, blood vessels, and ultimately every single cell of your body. You can concentrate on a large part of your body, such as all the muscles of your stomach area, or a tiny part of your body, such as the tip of your tongue.

Your conscious will allows you to send your attention anywhere inside your body, wherever you choose to direct it. And you can affect any part of your body from the inside.

You can wiggle your toes if you want to loosen their joints, or you can contract their muscles when you want to strengthen them.

Movement of body parts is not necessary for Extracise. Extracise is independent of external movements, but you can add it to any external exercise you desire.

Your conscious will is the director of your practice of Extracise. For example, you can sit on a chair and decide to contract you stomach muscles. You can do this anytime, anywhere, under most circumstances. In the same way, you can practice conscious breathing anytime, anywhere.

My Personal Experience Practicing Extracise

I love to move my body into various positions, breathe in and out, flex my muscles, breathe into and out of my muscles, be aware of tensions and pressures, gently rotate joints, increase blood circulation, increase energy circulation, bring clarity to my thinking mind through inner concentration, use my conscious will to sense my way into various muscle groups, listen to my heartbeat, observe my breathing; feel the tension in my muscles and tendons when I turn and twist my body, when I press my hands against the floor or a doorjamb, breathe into and out of muscles groups while using my conscious will to contract and relax them.

It's all about experiences, inner experiences, such as the breath flowing in and out, such as muscle contractions caused by my will. That's important to me. Inner experiences. "Extracise always! All the time!"

Listening to the sound of the incoming and outgoing breath. Paying attention to the still point in between them, when my head is quiet, all the noises stop, and stillness prevails for a while. Then the clear perception of the moment surfaces. When that happens, I feel as if I should just stop the breath and remain in this still awareness forever. But then the natural urge of the body for oxygen arises, and the activity continues.

The taste of this powerful still awareness lingers on and entices me return to it over and over again. Making a slight raspy sound with both incoming and outgoing breaths. I feel the sensation of bliss arise; "I am" "I am" "I am" "I exist."

I love doing the breathwork. I breathe into the individual muscles to exercise any and all of them. I breathe into the stomach area, biceps, feet, calves, buttocks, chest, stomach. I breathe into the power center, wherever I feel it. "I am breathing in – I am breathing out." I could add the mantra "So" on the outbreath and the mantra "Ham" on the inbreath. Perhaps add a slight raspy sound both times.

When contracting the muscles at will, without any other body movement, a certain load is placed on the heart, a resistance to the normal blood flow. So, the heart needs to work a little harder, which in turn exercises the heart muscles. This is similar to resistance training. Contracted muscles slow the blood flow and yet they also need more oxygen to burn fuel for the added activity (the contraction).

The breathwork: Breathe in – breathe out. It's easily done. It provides easy access to bliss and joy and pleasure. In freedom. In stillness. The best rest is in the Self, using the natural focus with the breath in the Self, in the "I am."

Take A Body Inventory

Before beginning your workout, first take inventory, investigate to see what you have to work with. Take your body for a little spin. Listen to it. Check it out. What are your capabilities and what are your limitations? What do you enjoy doing? Listen to your body, and also pay close attention to your mind and feelings.

Do some bends and twists, flex some muscles. See what condition your body is in. Just be an observer. Don't judge yourself against some model that you have heard about or seen. With model I mean not only an actual physical model, but also an ideal that you may have picked up some time somewhere about what your body should look like, or what your capabilities should be.

At this moment you are only concerned with finding out where you are at, what you have to work with.

After establishing your personal baseline, you will know what your body needs, where your focus should be, where you want to see improvements.

Where To Practice

Practice Extracise in a safe setting, where you can truly be yourself, can fully concentrate, and can go deeply into the awareness of your body.

It doesn't have to be complexly quiet. It should just be a safe space and an environment that you are comfortable in, where you can close your eyes and turn within.

Extracise does not lend itself to group practices with others, even close friends, because there is always an element of competition and comparison in groups. This will throw you off your personal game, even if just subtly. You need to pay attention only within, not without.

Everybody brings their own energy to the workout. You may have a need for quiet postures, while your friend is shifting back and forth.

So, your workout will rarely ever be in sync with someone else's. Any distraction of your game is a distraction and a deviation from your goal of really getting to know your body's inner workings.

The Need for A Purpose

There needs to be a sense of purpose to your practices, to the moving or the still forms you utilize to energize the muscles, the mind, the vital organs.

Vital energy must flow through the body and its organs for your body to function properly. Stagnation is the cause of imbalances, which will lead to health problems down the line.

Overdeveloped muscles will take on fat when not continually worked on. Stagnation is something that creeps in, slowly, and then nibbles away at your energy level.

Boredom is another reason to give up on your workout. More stimulation is **not** the key to keep you involved. More contentment and peace will do just nicely. More awareness of your inner health will keep you engaged, not outer stimulants from a trainer who yells at you and whips you into shape. No.

The search must always be for the inner glory. That will keep you motivated and enthralled.

Be wary of suppressing pain. Look at it, talk with it, let it tell you its secrets. Why is it there? What is it trying to tell you? What is its message to you?

Muscles cry out for help. Tendons don't want to be forced beyond their comfort zone. Joints can become loose or tight and tell you their level of mobility. Nerves get pinched and send out an alarm.

Always listen to your body, its parts, joints, muscles, nerves, tendons, ligaments, blood pressure, heart rate, level of wellbeing, feelings of hot or cold, being relaxed or frantic, experiencing stress or calm-abiding.

Are you expending more energy than you are taking in? Are you forcing your body to exert itself for some external goal? Are you in touch with your inner center, your personal rhythm? Do you know who you truly are? Are you following trends or are you forging your own path?

Personal Experiences

I have become a strong believer in breathing exercises, concentrated mental focus, and physical strengthening.

I have practiced all three continuously for many years now and I credit my good health with this practice. There are so many realizations I have had over the years practicing my form of health maintenance.

When I walk, I do what I call "Walking Out." I exaggerate the walking, consciously contracting various (otherwise unused) muscles, which increases the load on the heart and thereby Extracises the heart. While walking, I breathe consciously into the body activity, which keeps my thoughts to a minimum. This gives me a deep sense of presence and of peace. I look around and see beauty all around. I am aware of my surroundings. I sense the impact of my shoes on the ground and adjust it, so it is most comfortable and the least distracting. I keep my head up and my spine straight.

Talking about the spine: it is, besides the brain, the most important part of the body. All nerves run through it. According to the practice of Yoga, several vital energy centers reside in it. It is of the utmost important to keep the spine flexible, as well as erect. One of my secrets is that I breathe through the spine. That sounds a bit farfetched, but that is how it feels to me. I pull the energy up through the spine into my brain with the inbreath and let it flow downward with the outbreath. This gives me a slight ecstatic feeling and I sense a state of direct and deep presence.

Balance is another one of my interests. Performing physical movements evenly to the right and left sides of my body, as well as forward and backward. I stand on one leg for a while and then the other. I stand with my straight legs together, the knees and feet touching, while swaying my upper body to the left and right, twisting it left and right, bending it forward and backward. Always with the focus on the spine and the breathing. I turn my head left and right, up and down. All this with the emphasis on maintaining physical balance.

When balancing my body, I look for that sweet spot where I am able to relax as many muscles as possible and still maintain my posture. I sense a kind of weightlessness when I do that. This is quite a euphoric sensation to have.

Eye exercises are important to me. I stand or sit erect, looking straight ahead. Then I move one of my hands in wide circles while following it with my eyes without moving my head.

Sometimes I practice Jin Shin Jyutsu, a Japanese healing method. It balances the subtle energy body flow through the use of energy locks that are located at various areas of the body. These locks are similar to acupressure points. The hands touch the energy locks and the arms act as jumper cables to connect them. I do this practice at times while walking. It keeps me in focus and gives me a deep sense of physical and mental wellbeing. Jin Shin Jyutsu is called the art of knowing myself. It allows for my subtle energy to circulate within me. And: I balance the left and right side of my energy body in this very easy way.

I often hold my body positions for extended periods of time. I have learned that a good stretch requires at least fifteen seconds of staying in the same position.

On The Practice

I don't just practice Extracise during fixed times. I exercise various body parts during the times of the day when there are breaks in my activities. For example: I stand in line at the supermarket checkout, and I have time for some conscious breathing, as well as some subtle Extracises with my body. Perhaps I raise my body up on its toes, or I contract my chest or shoulder muscles. I may breathe into my arm muscles while contracting them gently. Or I tighten my stomach muscles while breathing in and out through my lower abdomen. Things like that. Consciously something extra.

Or I get tired of sitting in a waiting room and get up and walk down the hall, swinging my arms and performing my "walking out" routine. Or I get off my waiting room chair and stretch a bit while contracting various muscle groups together with consciously breathing into them.

I don't do distracting exercises of any kind while driving my car. It's too dangerous in this situation, unless I have stopped at a red light for a while and could use something to release some tension.

One of my basic tenets is that anything that I don't normally do can be called "workout," from the wiggling of my little finger to the lifting of a twenty-pound weight over my head.

Balance in life is important to me. This includes the balance of my physical body. Accidents can happen when people lose their balance while walking or standing. I do not do well with balancing my body when I wear my prescription eyeglasses. They tend to distort my sense of balance. That is why I am very careful when I climb a ladder or stool to change a light bulb. I take it one step at time, while holding on to something fixed to steady myself.

Many of the practices I do have the focus on balancing the body. I stand on one leg and swing the other vigorously to train myself to keep balance. I close my eyes to make this practice more challenging. To me, workouts are the preparation for eventual emergencies. I never know what is going to happen next in my life. I could trip over a crack in the sidewalk and have to catch my balance.

Once I drove my little razor scooter past an alley out of which came a large SUV that I had to avoid. I had to take a few large steps leaping through the air to regain my balance, while holding on to the scooter and the dog I was exercising at the time.

Nothing much happened, except for the look of a shocked SUV driver and my heart pounding for a while. I had the presence of thought to turn my head and smile reassuringly at her, to let her know, "no harm done."

My body was able to deal with this surprise situation. Without continuous preparation through daily exercises, the outcome could have been different. That is one of the reasons why I exercise regularly. I want to be ready for the unexpected emergency when it comes.

My blood pressure is pretty good. I just took it, and it was 111 over 74. The lower number is a bit high, but I think it is not too bad. I am not on any medication other than vitamin D3, about 2000 units per day. The only downside with my very good blood numbers is that I only visit a doctor once for my annual physical checkup. So, if anything more serious would suddenly pop up, I would not have much of a rapport with my internist.

My Spiritual Path

I started out as a catholic believer, moved into Greek and Roman philosophy; then, with the help of various Indian and Western gurus got into practices such as yoga, pranayama, and meditation; I had a powerful experience with the Hawaiian god Kuka Ilimoku; a personal experience with Jesus; a personal experience with YHWH; a personal interaction with the Greek god Zeus; I developed an affinity for the Koran and the Tibetan Book of the Dead; there was a Kalachakra Initiation by the Dalai Lama. And there have been several more spiritual connections to other influences as well.

I meditate on a variety of spiritual energies with the help of mantras and images. My favorite right now is Surya, the sun. I take the sun to be the true life giving and life supporting energy in my personal existence. Whenever I think of it, my mind gets lighter, and I feel freer and more peaceful. Tensions melt away and my awareness clears up.

I do not know exactly what will happen to my spirit after it leaves this body, but from what I have been reading in the Tibetan Book of the Dead and in Huna teachings, I have a pretty good idea that my physical death will not be the end of me.

On Pain

Now a few words about pain, mostly physical, but when it hits, it totally affects mind and spirit. Of course, I try to avoid pain, just like every other sane person would do, but I do not consider pain to be something to be avoided at all costs.

Pain in my knees, for example, tells me to be more careful when I exercise so as not to put too much strain and pressure on them.

When I have neck pain, I know that my posture may be off and that I need to take a time-out for a correction.

I once had a severe neck spasm where even the slightest movement caused my muscles to lock up and send me into an intense shock of pain. I realized that my muscles were telling me that they had been overworked and they were going on strike, therefore the spasm.

Movement of my head in any direction brought on this severe and debilitating neck spasm. Eventually I discovered that a soft neck brace allowed me to move my body slightly. Little by little I adjusted my position without causing the spasm and eventually I got through this excruciatingly painful episode. I realized that I had been sitting on my desk in an improper posture and had overused some of my neck muscles in the process. These muscles complained that they needed to be supported by other muscles around them. I found a way to do just that. It took several hours of slow exercise of my neck and spine to find the right balance. This was a great lesson. And the pain taught me where my improper physical alignment had been.

Another time I had the most excruciating headache, caused by aggravated sinuses from eating cold dairy products, combined with eyestrain from reading too much. Usually, two tablets of Tylenol deal with this kind of a problem, but not on that particular day. The pain was so intense that my body started shaking on its own. I thought of hitting my head against the wall to get some relief. For a while I used Reiki, a Japanese healing method, but it made me even more sensitive, and the pain increased. At some point I felt the Reiki energy suddenly shutting off by itself. That was unexpected. It had never happened before.

I realized there was no relief from my agony, as it went on unabated for several hours. That's when I adjusted my mental attitude towards the pain. I decided I needed to consider it my welcomed friend. I laid down on my bed and just experienced its full blast without fighting it. It was severe and my legs were shaking, but underneath the agony I sensed a calm bliss somewhere in the depth of my being. I began to consider this pain as another experience that I was going through. It was neither "good" nor "bad." It just "was." And on some level, it had become a part of me that I had learned to appreciate.

The lesson I learned from it? Avoid cold dairy and reading too much as a combination.

I know that there are basically two kinds of physical pain: nerve pain and muscle pain. Nerve pain responds to cold, while muscle pain responds to heat. The cold numbs the nerve, while the heat relaxes the muscle and increases the blood flow.

Muscles need to get warmed up before being used. One morning I walked around and stood barefoot on my cold kitchen floor for quite a while. Then I went for a jog around the neighborhood. When I came back, my Achilles tendons were so sensitive that I couldn't touch them, and they did not allow me to walk for a couple of days. I had done some light warm-ups, but not enough to loosen up my feet muscles and tendons after the exposure to the cold kitchen floor. An oversight on my part. Another lesson learned!

My Mornings and Evenings

Every morning I spend some time out on the balcony on a comfortable mat. I choose my Extracises depending how my body and mind feel on that day. Sometimes I do a lot of repetitions, almost interval training, and at other times I hold poses until my muscles begin to shake and it takes some effort to carefully get back into neutral territory. For many of my balancing exercises I close my eyes and find my center. It is liberating to close my eyes. There are trees in front of me and they are nice to look at, but I love my focus to be within.

After a combination of twists and turns, ups and downs, swinging of the arms, stretching of the spine, reversal of fluids, and vital energy movements combined with the conscious breath, I then sit cross-legged on the mat and allow for the energy to settle. I close my eyes and just be there. I stop my mind from thinking and focus on something higher, which is my sense of wellbeing and bliss. What more do I want? I am happy in the moment. Then some thoughts intrude, and I forget my serenity. After a while, the thought train stops, and I find myself wondering how I got on that train. Usually, it has to do with something I need to be doing or should have done already or something I am worrying about.

In the evening, right before going to bed, I practice Extracise for a few minutes. It helps me be more relaxed and it probably adds to my ability to fall asleep very fast.

The Phases Of The Breath

There are four phases to breathing. There is the in-breath, followed by a breath retention. Then there is the out-breath, also followed by a breath retention. Energy moves while the breath moves. When the breath stops, energy movement also stops. Through the moving breath you can move energy into any part of your body. For example: you consciously breathe in and with your will direct energy into your biceps, while simultaneously contracting your biceps. Then you hold the breath and the muscle contractions, all the while being aware the impact of this workout has on your body and sense of wellbeing. After a while you release the muscles and the breath.

Do this routine with all the muscles in your body. It gives you a certain amount of control over the breath as well as over your muscles, and it strengthens your willpower as well as your muscles, including the heart muscle. I personally like it when the heart has to push a little harder to get blood into my blood vessels through this intentional resistance exercise.

The Final Breath

The final breath is the last breath of a person. It is important to know how to breathe this final breath. It is important because it will determine the way you are transitioning out of this body.

The more attached you are to your body, your mind, and emotions, the more you will suffer at the end of your life. Lesser attachment leads to a lessening of this suffering. This lessening of attachment to body and mind can be achieved through drugs or through the natural means of the conscious breath.

Since the usage of drugs takes away your personal choice, you really should attempt to ease this transition by means of the conscious breath.

The practice of the conscious breath begins as soon as you decide it should begin. Do not wait too long to begin, because you do not know when the time of your final breath will be. The less practice you have, the less it will have the desired effect of lessening the pain of the separation of your life force from your body/mind system.

The conscious breath should be practiced every moment of your life without interruption. Through the practice of the conscious breath, you are connecting to the pure life force that is active inside of your body/mind system. By becoming aware of the existence of this life force that is the cause of your body/mind system you begin to shift your sense of identification away from body/mind and towards this pure life force.

Since all pain and suffering are only experienced in the body/mind system, the identification with the life force will result in a lessening of all pain and suffering of body/mind.

The same life force that enters you through your breath also enters you through the foods you eat and the liquids you drink. You could learn to focus on this life force instead of on the life force coming into your body through the breath. You could learn to focus on your last meal.

It is just that the breath goes on 24 hours a day, without interruption, while you only take in food and water 2-3 times a day.

Concentration on the breath can take place continuously without interruption, all day long. This is a very easy and very effective method of lessening your attachment to your body and mind. This will come in handy when you experience physical, mental or emotional hardships. The final moments of your life are likely to be a hardship to you. The conscious breath can help you at this time.

The final breath is actually a concept that has its origins in Yoga. When breathing in and out, the emphasis lies on giving up all attachments together with the breath.

The final breath is ultimately neither the breathing in, nor the breathing out, but the merging of the breath in the still state of breath that occurs between the in-and outbreath.

There are two still states: after breathing in and after breathing out. These states are called the states of breath retention.

Some breath exercises erroneously focus on bringing in positive energies with the inbreath and releasing negative energies with the outbreath. These exercises have nothing to do with the final breath concept. They only try to please the mind and body. They are not designed to give up attachment to body and mind.

Non-attachment to body and mind occurs naturally when your sense of identification shifts – through practice – from identification with body/mind to identification with the experience of the life force that moves with the breath.

In order to relinquish attachment to one thing, one must have something higher to focus on. The body/mind system is on a lower level than the life force, therefore attachment to body/mind is easy to overcome. You will become attached to the experience of the life force, but now you don't have the same problems as you had when you were attached to the body/mind system: In this life force there is no more sense of individuality, no more sense of time and space, no more sense of individual doership. In the experience of the lifeforce you are free of all limitations that were associated with the body/mind system.

You will truly swim in an ocean of ecstasy, free from the shackles of physical and mental restrictions. Before, you were separated from all other living and not-living things, but now you feel and see yourself as one with them and as part of the freely existing life force in existence.

This is the result of the practice of the final breath. Every breath is potentially your final breath. Therefore, every breath should be taken in a conscious manner. Be aware of it, listen to it, feel it, merge with it, identify with it. This practice will allow you to let go of identification with body and mind. You know that the final breath will come to you eventually. Breathe consciously into and out of the still space between the in- and outbreath and experience contentment.

The State Of Magnificence

To get into a state of extended magnificence, find something that evokes a sense of wonder in you. This "something" can be anything, from a photo to a live sunset, from a rock to a diamond, from an insect to a whale. There is nothing that is not appropriate for this exercise.

Once you sense the magnificence, then remain in this state until it fills you completely, until your mind and entire being are completely saturated by it. This state is the most valuable state to be in. Whenever you are given a chance to be in this state, remain in it indefinitely.

At times, this sense of magnificence comes unexpectedly during your everyday activities. Don't reject this gift at that moment. Enjoy it fully and be thankful for the opportunity.

Awareness

The easy act of shifting your attention to your breathing brings about a greater awareness of your entire body/mind system, because the state of your breath can tell you a lot about the state of your body and your mind. Are you uptight and agitated? Are you relaxed and collected?

You should always look for clarity in your thoughts and feelings, as well as in your body. "Do I feel any resentment towards anyone at the moment?" "How does this resentment manifest in my body"?

"Do I sit/stand/lie properly so that the life-energies can flow unimpededly through my body?"

"Is there something that I am neglecting in my life that needs to be taken care of?" "How does that knowledge affect my practice of Extracise?" Etc.

First comes breath, then other things. Breath is the best indicator of your mental state. Agitated breath leads to agitated thinking and agitated doing. Relaxed breathing equals relaxed thinking and relaxed acting.

The body always tells the truth. You cannot hide from its truth. You are either at peace with yourself and your surroundings, or you are not. The body knows. You can tap into its awareness for a greater understanding of your state of being.

Meditate On Bliss

Meditation on Bliss is the natural way to establish it within your being. Meditation does not require a lot of paraphernalia to be effective. Meditation does not require a special place or time for its benefits to appear. Meditation can happen right here, right now. All you need for the practice is you, the way you are right now. There is no need for breathing exercises or physical adjustments. What is called "asana" is simply a physical pose that makes it possible for you to remain comfortably and indefinitely in the state of meditation.

Always strive toward the more blissful. That is the only criteria on the spiritual path.

The Body Speaks To You

When your joints are beginning to ache as a result of sitting for quite some time, I suggest doing a few moving forms to loosen up, while simultaneously energizing yourself. Consciously breathe into the joint movements and the associated stretches. This will make you feel better, more balanced, as well as relaxed and vitalized.

The greatest benefits await you when you are doing your Extracises in a very attentive way. There is much to be gained from conscious and focused breathing in conjunction with balancing postures.

Sometimes during your practice, you may have a sense of expanded space inside you. This experience is very peaceful and relaxing.

When doing an exercise that causes pain in you, look carefully at what it is your doing and adjust your workout. Don't push through the discomfort.

If you do not listen to your body and are overextending yourself and as a result begin to suffer from some debilitation, then you are not practicing Extracise. It is important that you closely monitor your own actions and do not push yourself through any pain barrier. It is solely your responsibility to carefully monitor yourself with a sort of feed-back loop in order to truly benefit from your workouts.

While standing and twisting your body, always protect your knee joints by either slightly bending your knees, or by stiffening them – locking them.

Do some of your Extracises with a gently swaying motion fully conjoined with the conscious breath.

In the morning, perform vertical poses. Those are good for deeper inhalation and exhalation. In the evening, perform horizontal poses. Those are more balancing and relaxing. During the day, perform poses that feel right at that moment and are appropriate to your environment.

For some balancing standing poses, put your feet and knees together, close your eyes, and gently move the upper body, swing the arms, twist upper body, raise arms, bend your hips gently to the left – right, forward – backward, turn head to the left – right – down – back. If there is pressure on the knees, relax them slightly.

Arms stretched out sideways in 3/9 o'clock position. Alternate between positions upwards 12 o'clock – sideways 3/9 o'clock – downwards 6 o'clock.

Keep feet and knees together. Swing both arms in wide circles from the 12 o'clock to the 6 o'clock position while bending at the hip and coming as close as easily possible to touching the ground. This large oval is your sphere of influence. Combine this exercise with your incoming and outgoing breath.

If your mouth gets dry, take small sips of plain water, nothing stimulating!

Struggling to maintain your physical balance is part of the effort. It prepares your body for emergencies. If you consistently lose your balance with eyes closed, then open them slightly.

While standing erect, lower your arms and place your hands on the ground with your legs as straight as possible without straining. Gently rocking forward and backward, shifting your weight from the hands to the feet, raising up on your toes. Gently swaying side to side, stretching your back in concert with your breathing. Perhaps some walking forward and backward, like a bear.

Some movement of the body is necessary to help with the moving of the waste products through and out of the body, to keep the joints and tendons flexible, and to be able to maintain a healthy overall physical balance.

Much of the benefits of physical workouts comes in handy during emergency situations, such as tripping, stumbling, falling, mis-stepping, getting pushed or shoved, etc. Those are the times when your body needs to spontaneously react to a sudden and unexpected, and potentially harmful event.

Personal Experiences

As a kid, I enjoyed a particular calming body pose, where I laid on my back with the legs over my head and the knees touching the ground next to my ears. Every time my mother saw me like that, she told me to join the local gymnastic team. I had no interest in them, because I did not think they were doing the kind of exercises that I really wanted to do. Later I found that this particular posture is called "the spider" in Hatha Yoga. It is a variation of the "the plow" asana. Doing it felt very relaxing to me, and it still does today.

One of my earlier memories as a child of about twelve or thirteen has to do with me lying in bed and staring at a small spot on the wall for as long as could. I don't know what possessed me, but I felt drawn to do it. My eyes would start to burn and get very watery, but I kept at it. After looking at the spot for a while, my mental focus became stronger and stronger, and my peripheral vision began to shrink more and more. I loved the feeling of concentrated attention and practiced it whenever I thought about it.

One night, I had a dream in which I felt very, very small and concentrated, like the size of a single atom, while simultaneously feeling as expanded as the whole universe. This was a great and blissful feeling, and I loved it. When I woke up, I felt truly alive and conscious.

Paying Attention

Throughout the day, pay attention to the messages of your body. Are there tensions, pains, or discomforts? Immediately attempt to find a remedy or stop the activity until you have more time to investigate.

Don't push through pain. Don't ignore it. If you must – as a temporary solution – take a pain pill, so be it, but don't keep using this as your only solution to the discomfort. The next time it happens, take your time to find a more permanent and drug-free solution.

Talk to an expert, get a second opinion, do your own research. It's your body, your health, that's at stake. You want to live in your body pain free and in comfort until a ripe old age. Resources to assist you are always available. Don't be shy to ask for help. Don't ignore unpleasant symptoms for too long. A problem avoided is NOT a problem solved.

As you are advised in pain management after a surgery. "Stay ahead of the pain. Don't chase it." The same is true with health: "Stay ahead of health." Meaning: "Stay healthy. Don't chase health after problems develop."

During rehab after a surgery or an accident, you will have to go through several layers of pain and discomfort before your body settles into the state of a "new normal." Be as fully conscious of all aspects of your rehab as possible. Don't fight against the process. Sink into your stretches with the outgoing breath, fully aware of the discomfort you are experiencing. Contract your muscles with the help of your conscious will. See where your limitations are and accept them, while consciously striving to overcome them. Find a way to consider the at times considerable pain to be your best friend on the road to recovery. Don't hate it. Like everything else in life – including life itself – it is a gift.

A Breathing Practice

Breathe in and out through the nostrils, into a singular spot inside your brain. That spot is where your conscious self resides. The conscious will, which is a part of you, is concentrating your attention there. You are concentrating on yourself, your conscious being. You have crept out of the fog of unconsciousness and now you are self-aware, conscious, in the single point of breathing in and out.

There is no external focus. It is all internal. As a consequence, everything merges within you and there is only the "I am" consciousness. "I am alive." "I am." "I exist."

It is important to do this exercise in a state of complete relaxation and openness. Let the experience come to you. Never chase this or any other experience. Always let all experiences come to you. Let them unfold within you. Don't force them. Don't add to them with help from your memory. You never know how any experience will unfold, what it will tell you, what you will experience.

In that sense, all experiences are new experiences on the road of life. They are never exactly the same, even if they start out appearing the same.

All our lives started in pretty much the same fashion: we came through a birth canal. After that, we went in our different directions.

It is the same with all experiences. You may sit here, day after day, at the same time, and do the same breathing exercise, but there are differences in how these breaths unfold. Be aware of it. At some point, tears will well up inside of you over the exquisite beauty of this world, this existence, your existence, the existence of all there is.

Where To Focus During The Practice

The focus is always within. Your will directs it there. Outer forms of body movements follow from this call of the interior, towards the interior. In the interior is where you are truly you. This is where your most authentic self resides. Outer body forms are not where your focus should lie.

When you raise your arm, the focus should be on the awareness of raising it – the awareness and the will of contracting the muscles – then releasing them with your will and awareness – being fully conscious that all this activity is taking place within you, within your being, within your existence.

Feelings of wellbeing spread through your body as a result of your body movements and muscular contractions-relaxations. Your efforts should never be harsh, but always gentle and considerate.

Perceive your body to be an extension of yourself. It is precious, because you are precious.

Focus on the preciousness of your existence. Breathe in and out from a center of preciousness. Be fully aware, fully conscious.

Keep your eyes closed to maintain your inner focus. This will prevent you from getting pulled towards an outer focus. Listen within and go deeper and deeper into the stillness and peace that reside at your inner core.

At first, it may be a bit lonely in your center, devoid of all others, of all subjects-objects to focus on, but once you touch your inner core – your inner sense of being – you will be satisfied to the point of tears welling up inside of you at the realization of the beauty that you truly are. The outer points-of-interests then fade away like shadows, and you stand-sit-lie in your own living beauty and exquisiteness. You have descended into the sizzling world of blissful consciousness.

And yes, there is love for what you do, for what your body tells you, for the awareness you are experiencing, for the sense of being alive, of existing.

The emphasis is always within, finding that sweet balance of comfort-ease and the purposefully directed will of your conscious efforts. That is the art of being and the science of living. Your body and mind will thank you for experiencing it.

Here is a question for you: Who is setting your personal exercise goals? Are you truly free from external influences in your practice of physical cultivation? What are your expectations, your markers of success? Who or what do you measure yourself up to? Another person? A certain number of repetitions? A particular timespan? A milestone? Something that someone else at some point has placed as their marker? The highest? The fastest? The best in comparison with whom or what?

Today is today. This moment is this moment.

One of my slogans is: "Live like there is no tomorrow, and work like there was no yesterday."

Don't rest on your laurels, your achievements from yesterday. They mean nothing anymore. Always make the best efforts when dealing with the present. Be most attentive to all nuances of your body, breath, and mind.

Always go for the extra mile, towards the essence within your experiences. That's the only way to truly understand your body and to control your sense of wellbeing in this magnificent nine-gated city. Make truly peace with your body, breath, and mind.

Thoughts On Walking, Jogging, and Running

My way of getting into walking, jogging, or running may sound a bit strange, but it works for me and has brought me to extended states of blissful inner stillness.

I start in a relaxed standing position. Then I lean forward until I begin to feel that I am losing my balance. That is when my legs – quite automatically – begin to move, to prevent me from falling forward (and from hitting the ground).

The further I lean forward, the faster my legs have to move to keep up. I then find myself in a state of balance, where I feel as if I am continuously falling, pulled by the force of gravity, while experiencing a kind of weightlessness and stillness of mind. I keep looking to the ground for obstacles while I "fall along."

This practice is similar to the movement of a spaceship orbiting the earth. Gravity is constantly pulling the spaceship towards the earth, but the speed of the craft is so great that it keeps missing the earth. And so, it keeps falling around the earth.

I have been experiencing deep inner peace and contentment while I practice this form of walking, jogging, or running. I feel weightless and timeless and spaceless in this state of continually falling forward.

Mobility And Flexibility

Mobility comes with flexibility. Check out the range of your mobility from whatever body position you are in, (lying, sitting, standing, squatting, etc.), and gently extend it. Do this with your arms, fingers, legs, torso, neck and shoulders, knees, feet, hips, jaw, ears, eyes, nose, tongue, mouth, cheeks.

Make an inventory of your body parts and consciously work on them with the focus on inner wellbeing. While you are twisting and bending your upper body, remember that you are also massaging your inner organs, your heart, lungs, etc. including your intestines.

Lean your head back to drain your sinuses.

Begin with the area of greatest needs, then expand your efforts. Don't neglect your toes and fingers, eyelids, mouth, tongue, and all the muscles of your face and head.

You are consciously working on every muscle, joint, and tendon of your body. You can do that either systematically, starting with your toes and ending with your head, or you can begin where you feel the greatest need and focus on that first, and then go to the next area that needs it, and so on, until you have completed your entire body.

There may be problem areas, such as neck and shoulders, or the hands, or the back, that you always want to make sure you work on, even if you have limited time available. You get these problematic or sensitive areas out of the way first, and then move on to the rest of your body.

Always be especially careful with your knees when rotating your body.

Don't do your Extracises automatically, without a sense of purpose or without paying close attention. Do them with reverence, even with a sense of holiness – of divinity.

During your practice, whatever contorted shape you twist yourself into, however long you are holding a pose, remember that you will need some strength to straighten yourself out again.

Also practice some eye circles, where your open eyes follow the wide circles of your hands without moving the head. Bring the hands closer to the eyes to work on the muscles that pull and contract your lenses. Often times we focus for a long period of time on one distance, a computer monitor for example, or on the little smartphone screen in our hands. This exhausts those eye muscles and makes them inflexible over time.

Consciously move the joints of your fingers, until you feel the muscles in the fingers. Feel the warm comfort from those energized muscles. When was the last time you felt the muscles in your little fingers? Don't' forget to consciously breathe into your muscle contractions and joint movements.

About The Workout

You can perform your workouts by either holding forms or by repeating them. As an example: You can perform twenty sets of the Yoga sequence "Salutations to the Sun" in twenty minutes by moving continuously, or you can perform one set in twenty minutes by holding the individual poses longer. It is up to you, but the focus must always be within, at the center of your being, at your still point, with an awareness of the impact of your forms on all parts of your body and your mind. You will fall in love with your body while doing these very personal workouts, while getting to know your body intimately from head to toe.

Another helpful set of exercises comes from Chi Kung. It is called "The Eight Pieces of Brocade." These pieces are a good starting point for your Extracise practice.

Make use of the natural force of gravity to assist you in your workouts. Let it pull you when you are bending your body and push against it when you straighten your body. Do this with full awareness while you breathe into and out of the movements.

When you encounter a weakness or a pain during your workout, stop what you were doing and see if you can find a way through or around the problem area, slowly and deliberately, carefully. Gently move your body and see where the limitation begins and where it ends. Then circle around it with your full attention and see if you can make the area of discomfort smaller. Define it as much as possible. Let the discomfort be your indicator and guide.

Always love what you do during Extracise, never dislike, or hate anything you come across while practicing. Accept limitations, appreciate them, and then see if you can move around them or through them, while still honoring them and regarding them as your guide forward towards optimal health.

When you are too stiff or lack energy one morning, don't force your body into doing what it does not want to do. Pay close attention and listen to your body. Perhaps the problem does not reside in this moment, but further back, perhaps yesterday, when you did something to overburden your system, and now you can't fully commit to your workout.

Ask yourself: "What can I do in my present state?" That should be your only concern. Listen to your body. Then act. Whatever you do, always do it with your full attention, full concentration, full conscious will, even if you only have a few minutes to wake up your body and get it energized. Perhaps you only have time for a couple of deep breaths combined with some muscle contractions. Make those count! Do them fully and consciously. That will wake you up and get you going.

Whenever doing any kind of workout involving the knees, see if you can distribute your weight evenly between both knees, not favoring one over the other too much. Stay away from extreme deep knee bends using only one knee.

If you ever come across muscle cramps, stop what you are doing and let them pass. Don't hate them. They are indicators that you have overburdened a muscle. If they are severe, massage the area and relax your muscles, tendons, and joints, while breathing into them. Always honor your body.

Use Of A Mantra

If you want to use a mantra or a power word to add to your sense of inner strength, consciously use the name "Sun." The Sun is the most powerful force in our immediate existence. It radiates unimaginable power.

We have seen it up there in the sky, moving slowly from east to west, since we were kids, but don't really pay much attention to it. It is just "up there," lighting our world.

In reality, it represents unimaginable forces, pure light, pure radiance, pure power. It is the true life-giving energy in our existence.

When you do your flex workouts, think of the wind flowing, moving gracefully, elegantly. Wind is pure flexibility. The inner wind is driving your outer forms.

About Reversal Of The Fluids

Something else that I find of excellent value is the reversal of fluids in the body. I accomplish this mostly by standing straight, raising my hands above my head, holding this form for a while, and then bending forward at the hip, allowing my arms to dangle in front of me until my hands slightly touch the floor.

Let gravity do the work and pull you down, slowly relaxing as many muscles as possible and breathing into the downward pull.

Remain in this position for about a thirty seconds to start with, and then slowly, in a sweeping motion straighten your torso and return to your starting position with arms pointing upwards. Don't straighten up too quick, or the blood may shoot up into your head and then gush back down again, which can make you feel dizzy, and you may lose your balance, especially if your eyes are closed!

Remain in this standing position for at least one minute. Sense how the fluid is draining from your arms.

Another way of reversing some of the body fluids is by lying on your back in a relaxed way, with the head resting on the floor and going into an easy shoulder stand. Relax all unneeded arm and leg muscles so you don't restrict the flow. Let your muscles enjoy their freedom in relaxation. Find that sweet spot where you are in perfect balance while only using the few muscles absolutely necessary to keep you in the upright position. Hold until you feel the fluids drain from your limbs. Then slowly lower the legs and arms and roll out your spine.

If a shoulder stand is not an option for you, then simply lie comfortably on your back and raise your arms and legs so they are pointing straight up. Relax your shoulders and all muscles not needed to hold this easier position. You could also rest your legs on a chair if that is more suitable for you, as long as they are higher than your heart.

This reversal of inner body fluids is important to me. I like to practice it in the morning as part of my workout. It is a very simple process. This reversal of fluids forces the arterial arteries to find a different way to distribute the blood throughout the body. It exercises these arterial muscles.

Get into these reversal positions carefully, slowly, and with full attention. If you feel discomfort of any kind, such as dizziness, pressure in your head, stop, and investigate.

You can add another benefit to the shoulder stand. Keep your ankles and knees together while you have your legs up in the air. Place your hands on top of your hipbones. There are energy meridian points in your ankles, your knees, and your upper hipbones. Touching them in this way balances the right and left energy flow of your body.

The shoulder stand could also become one of your Extracise starting positions. From here, explore which joints you can move, what muscles you can contract and relax, and which tendons you can stretch. Investigate, look around your body and see what you come up with while in this starting pose.

General Guidelines On Positions

Whatever position that you are in, relax all the muscles you don't need for that position. Then, as an added workout, consciously contract and relax those unneeded muscles, while deeply breathing into them on the contractions.

On the flip side, you can also become fully aware of the muscles that you do need for the particular body position, and consciously contract them a bit more than needed, while deeply breathing into the contraction.

Your focus should always be deep within yourself. You are entering your body with your mind fully aware of every nuance of your workout. Following your breath into the muscles, joints, and tendons gives you this ability.

An interesting way of breathing in and out is by slightly constriction your airways in your throat and thereby creating an almost raspy sound you can easily concentrate on.

Your Personal Practice

Your Extracise workouts will vary from those of other people, based on your knowledge of your body, your exercise history, your flexibility, your proclivities, your limitations and strengths, etc.

Also, when it's cold, you may want to practice more moving forms, to keep your body and muscles and joints and tendons warm and pliable.

When it's hot, perhaps more still forms or easy stretches feel better. Whatever needs your body has, that is exactly what you should pursue.

Don't tell yourself, "I am going to make up for a shortened practice of Extracise the next time." How do you know the next time will be a better time? Now is the important time. Do the best in the now with what you have. Be fully conscious, breathe, contract a muscle, move a joint, and stretch a tendon. If you can only do one Extracise, do it as fully in the moment — with as much attention and conscious will – as possible. Be the action!

I have been asked how long an Extracise session should last. Ideally, you should practice until you sense that your whole body has been invigorated and that you feel great inside your skin.

For maintenance, probably fifteen to twenty minutes once a day could be sufficient. For a deeper practice about thirty to forty-five minutes.

But you also should be doing some exercises during the day when you get a chance, to keep up the momentum. Always look for those moments when you add something extra to your normal routine.

I am not the "weekend warrior" type person, who is lazy all week and then exerts himself for a couple of days. That's also not what Extracise is all about.

Thoughts On Using Weights And TRX Straps

If you feel like using free weights to add to your workout, be aware that it is difficult to completely relax your muscles after contractions, because some muscles will always be required to hold the weights in your hands. Relax as many muscles as possible that are not associated with your workout.

If you feel like using the popular TRX straps, then relax your muscles as much as possible between your various moves. Also, locate those muscles you need for your moves and relax all other muscles not needed to practice them.

I like to completely relax my muscles between contractions. The idea is to start a muscle contraction at zero, bring it to my personal max, and then return it to zero.

At the end of your practice, bring all your muscles to zero, to complete relaxation, to complete inner relaxed and peaceful bliss.

A Personal Experience

A while ago I developed some pain in my shoulder. This started as a very slight discomfort and over many months became more noticeable and painful. For the longest time I couldn't figure out what was causing it. I tried to balance my workload between both shoulders, to no avail. Then, finally it dawned on me what could be the culprit. I was using a retractable leash when walking my dog for between thirty minutes to an hour. There was a constant slight pull on one of my shoulder muscles. I switched to a fixed leash and within days, the pain subsided and never returned. Who would have thought that this handy leash could create a shoulder problem? I figured it out because I took the time to pay close attention to my body. How many people would perhaps go to a physical specialist and ask them for help? And how many of those would suggest switching a dog leash?

I am mentioning this episode, because it shows how important it is to pay the closest attention to problems that arise in your body, especially over a long period of time.

Another example is similarly banal. One of my hamstrings was not as stretched out as the other. This was noticeable when I sat in a cross-legged position during meditation. It kept bothering me and I tried to remedy this by extra stretching right before crossing the legs. It helped a bit but did not solve the underlying cause.

Then, after months, I finally realized the cause: when I put on my pants while standing up, I raised one of my legs a bit higher than the other in order to step into the pant leg. And over time, this slight discrepancy caused the muscle to be more stretched out than the other. How to correct it? Alternating the legs when I put on my pants.

These examples show that even little things — seemingly insignificant — have an impact on the quality of my life.

On The Health Industry

There is a large industry that has sprung up around the subject of health and exercise. Companies sell everything from socks, to shoes, to clothing, to exercise machines, to wrist meters. A lot of these things are unnecessary. Yes, this book I am selling is part of this industry. I am hoping to free you from many of the externals that may clutter up your life and your mind.

My question about the necessity of things always comes down to this: "if I were stranded on a desert island, how would I get along without all these accoutrements?"

Another question that I tend to ask myself is: "how portable is my physical workout? How much room do I need? Where can I practice? What do I need to practice?"

I find that the less I need, the more likely it is that I practice my workouts. If I have to drive for fifteen minutes to get to a studio, then by the time I get there, I may have lost my verve. And then it's another fifteen minutes to get back home. That's thirty minutes I could have been doing already a sensible workout in my apartment.

I have always attempted to find my own way, away from the established crowd. And perhaps I am just reinventing the wheel with this practice of Extracise, although I find it invigorating and valuable. I love doing it. It has provided me with many hours of blissful interaction with my own body, doing the things that my body and mind enjoy. It's been truly blissful and a blessing. And I am deeply grateful for having found my way into it.

Thoughts On Inner Functions Vs. Outer Forms

During exercise, most people tend to focus on externals, such as the number of repetitions of a moving form (let's say twenty pushups, or ten knee bends, etc.), or the time spent working out (e.g., fifteen minutes on a treadmill, or a half hour jog through the neighborhood), while checking the heartrate with the help of a monitor (smartphone, etc.).

When doing Extracises, you may be doing pushups, or knee bends, or spending time on a treadmill, or jogging, but the focus would not be on external measurements to determine your state of health and wellbeing.

For example: Instead of doing the twenty pushups, you could in the same timeframe do only one extremely slow pushup with total concentration and awareness of the muscle, joint, and tendon action.

The conscious focus would only be internally, on the workings of your body, combined with breathing in a fully conscious way. And you are doing it mostly with your eyes closed so that you can concentrate better and more deeply.

The aim of the Extracise program is always to consciously bend or rotate every joint, fully contract and relax every muscle, fully stretch every muscle and tendon.

And you are doing it in concert with your directed breath and your conscious will, with a glad heart and mind.

Find your personal way of liberating yourself from any fixed form, whether you are standing, sitting, upside down, right side up, or whatever. Begin with a form, then explore from there. See where your body can take you. Be invigorated by your free forms.

Some Basic Extracise Starting Positions

The body is the tool. The conscious will is the driving force. The breath is the key.

You can begin your Extracise practice from any body position. Sit, stand, lay on your back, on your belly; crouch, kneel, on all fours, or whatever.

Any and all positions are perfect to begin your practice. To assist you I am suggesting six basic starting positions from which you can easily begin your practices.

Basic vertical starting position:

Standing erect, with feet comfortably apart and arms hanging by your sides.

Basic vertical starting position:

Standing erect, with feet comfortably apart, arms left and right horizontally, like a cross.

Basic vertical starting position:

Standing with feet comfortably apart, bent at the hip, with hands on the floor, distributing the weight evenly between the legs and the arms.

Basic horizontal starting position:

Sitting on the floor with your legs stretched out. Upper body is vertical, slightly leaning back with your straight arms behind it on the floor supporting some weight.

Basic horizontal starting position:

Laying on your back, with your arms stretched out on the floor over your head.

Basic horizontal starting position:

Your knees and hands are on the ground, with the legs and arms supporting the body.

Basic horizontal starting position:

Your knees and elbows are on the ground. There is a straight line that gets formed by your upper legs and your back, up to your neck. Your legs and elbows are supporting your weight.

Basic mixed starting position:

Sitting on your knees, your upper body is slightly leaning back with your straight arms behind it on the floor, with the body weight evenly distributed between your legs and arms.

Practice:

If you don't know what to do next in your practice of Extracise, remember that you want to fully bend or rotate all your joints, fully contract and relax all your muscles, and fully stretch all your muscles and tendons, using your conscious will. You are also simultaneously breathing into your muscle contractions and relaxations and joint movements and tendon stretches. And you are fully aware of your actions on the state of your body and mind.

That is always your overall mission. Execute the mission as a newborn baby explores their new body. With a sense of wonder and curiosity.

Take a little sip of water before your practice. Then relax and orient yourself inside your body.

Listen within the body. What does it want or need from you right now to feel better, more at ease, more vital, more alert, more at peace?

From your starting position, with a mental attitude of gratitude and appreciation, look around your body and determine what movement to do next. What part of your body is asking for – is demanding – your attention?

During your relaxed exercises, breathe only in and out through your nose. If your body needs more oxygen and more power during more vigorous movements, you can breathe in and out of your mouth, or do a combination of inbreath through the nose and outbreath through the mouth. Perhaps blowing the breath out through pursed lips.

While standing in a relaxed way, lift one leg off the ground. How is your balance? If you can, keep your eyes closed during your workouts and focus your attention deep inwards on your center.

Keep the spine flexible and stretched out, relaxed, but strong. Twist, turn, stretch. Lay on the floor. Roll backwards – forwards – sideways.

Breathe deeply into and out of your moves, always focusing on the inner center of perpetual stillness.

Here are a couple of basic assignments for you: wake up your body tomorrow morning for an energized day ahead and ease its transition in the evening for a restful sleep.

A Sample Extracise Session

Stand in the simple cross position, with your feet about a foot apart, and your arms stretched out horizontally to your sides.

Use your conscious will and contract the muscles in your hand, fingers, and lower arm muscles of one arm while breathing into them, without moving them. Hold for a few moments. Then breathe out and release the muscles. Repeat with the other arm, then repeat with both arms.

Use your conscious will and contract your upper arm muscles while breathing into them. Hold for a few moments. Relax them while breathing out. Repeat with the other arm, then repeat with both arms.

Use you conscious will and contract your shoulder muscles while breathing into them. Hold for a few moments. Then relax the muscles. Repeat with the other shoulder, then repeat with both shoulders.

Sense the stillness and invigoration at the end of each muscle relaxation. Always use your fully conscious will in your efforts, but never strain.

These exercises will help you get in touch with the individual muscles and muscle groups in your shoulders, arms, hands, and fingers.

Another simple pose:

Stand with your feet a bit apart. Slightly bend your knees.

Use your conscious will and contract the muscles in your toes, feet, and calves of one leg, while consciously breathing into them. Hold for a bit. Relax them while breathing out. Repeat with the other leg, then repeat with both legs.

Use your conscious will and contract the muscles in the thigh of one leg, while consciously breathing into them. Hold for a bit. Relax them while breathing out. Repeat with the other leg, then repeat with both legs.

Perform this contracting and breathing exercise with your buttocks, left and right. Then up into your lower stomach and upper stomach area. Then into your back. Then into your neck.

The more you practice with attention, the better you'll get at gaining access to individual muscles and muscle groups.

Now pay attention to your face. There are many muscles in it, and it seems impossible to control them all. Some people are afraid to exercise the face because they are worried about possible lines or creases that may develop. Well, sagging muscles do nothing to improve anyone's looks.

So, go over all the muscles in your face, but don't look in mirror while doing this, you might give up for looking "ridiculous". It's best to keep your eyes closed while doing this practice.

Wiggle your nose like Jeanie. Raise your eyebrows. Pucker your lips and stretch out your tongue. Pull up your cheeks. Move your ears. Lower and raise you jaw.

After a short while, your face will feel invigorated from the fresh blood flow this activity has generated. In fact, this practice could be done at the end of your overall workout to finish it all off, much like the icing on the cake.

The more you practice, the more you will get the hang of it.

Thoughts On The Practice

When starting your routine, take a few conscious breaths to get centered.

Get into an Extracise position with purpose, and then begin, moving, swaying, stretching your whole body.

Check out the mobility of every limb, every finger, every toe, and see if you can extend their mobility through conscious stretching while breathing into the stretch.

You may begin with your toes, then the feet and ankles. Move them in as many different directions as you can think of while consciously breathing into them. Then on to your knees. Avoid twisting them too much.

It's best to keep your eyes closed to concentrate fully on the inner effect and the inner needs of your body-mind. Fully listen inwardly, being fully aware.

Deeply experience the joy and invigoration of moving your body, of stretching your limbs, of flexing your muscles.

When you hold a position for a while, consciously breathe into the contracted muscles, the stretched tendons, the joints.

I'd suggest working on your neck, head and face last. Flexing your face muscles gives a nice warm invigorated feeling at the end of your workout.

Feel how this facial routine stimulates the blood flow, while strengthening the face and head muscles.

Towards the end of your routine, go mentally over every part of your body and feel how it is doing.

The harmony between all body parts is the result of having invigorated and worked over all parts evenly.

At the end of your workout, say "Thank You" to your body and mind, to all muscles, joints, and tendons, and to your brain, your awareness, and your consciousness.

Also say "Thank You" for being here on this plane of this existence. In other words, be reverential.

Just because you are doing a routine day after day does not mean it can't be fun. Enjoy each routine as if it were brand new, on a brand-new day, which it actually is! "Joie de vivre". Joy of living!

Joy of movement! Joy of breathing! Joy of existing! Joy of being here!

More On Pain

The sensation of pain is a message from your body that you must listen to. It's telling you that something is going on in your body that requests your immediate attention.

If you experience some pain when contracting a muscle, relax it and massage it gently, slowly digging deeper into it, in a circular way, then try again contracting it. If, after several attempt at loosening up the muscle fibers the pain persists, give up for now and move on to a different area of the body.

But, come back to this area of discomfort several times during your workout, to see if anything has changed. Or you can get back to it as the last exercise during your practice.

When you start a new workout, the first area to investigate would be any problem area that you discovered during your last workout. See where it's at. If it got worse, leave it alone for now. If it got better, see if you can gently work to completely eliminate it.

You could also do some slight tapping with your hands or fingers to stimulate a problematic muscle or tendon. You can do this tapping to increase the blood flow, or to entangle some stuck muscle fibers, or to free a stuck nerve.

At the end of your workout, you can do a little shaking out of the limbs to move the energy around, in case it had become a bit stagnant because you concentrated yourself into a piece of petrified wood.

Also, end your routine with some sense of gratitude for life having given you this body, mind, and spirit.

The truly scare fact about life is not that you will die one day, but that you have been and will continue to be part of this existence for eternity. And that thought can be truly overwhelming.

Yes, it's a bit scary to realize that you will be in existence forever. But you can't change that. You can't close your mind to this fact. You are here to stay!

The Conscious Will

Use the conscious will to move, bend, stretch, and breathe. Get away from the idea that "you" are doing this. Get into the idea of "there is movement," "there is bending," "there is stretching," "there is breathing."

This mindset leads to mental-emotional freedom and then there is the liberation in the experience of calm-abiding and resigned determination.

The conscious will is the key to a successful Extracise practice!

On Perfection

Always do the Extracise workouts with a sense of perfection. You are perfect. This moment is perfect. The movement is perfect. This posture is perfect. The breathing is perfect.

Don't do these exercises with a sense of pride over what you have accomplished. Perfection and pride may appear very similar, but in practice they are distant cousins. You want perfection, not pride.

At the end of your workout, look around inside your body and listen and feel if there is any area that you missed or neglected, that needs a bit more attention. Then go there and give it the attention it needs and wants.

About Food And Drinks

Eat only when you are hungry. Learn to distinguish between hunger pains and carb cravings.

Stop eating when you are satiated. Do not stuff yourself out of boredom, nervousness, or anxiety.

Be calm and confident in social situations where eating and drinking are encouraged. Peer pressure often pushes you into making decisions that do not line up with the true path of your body.

Think about the foods and drinks and other substances you're imbibing. Be aware of their effect on your sense of wellbeing, your sense of focus and purpose.

The choice is always going to yours; but you'll have to live with the consequences of your actions.

That's all I am going to say about this subject.

Extracise Highlights

At any given moment during you daily hours, ask yourself how to follow through on the Extracise mission of fully stretching all tendons and muscles, fully flexing all muscles, fully moving all joints, while using your conscious will to send vital energy to them through your breath.

Think about what Extracise practices you could do right now, right here.

Are you sitting? You can exercise your toes, feet, ankles, calves, knees, thighs, buttocks, stomach, chest, fingers, hands, lower and upper arms, shoulders, back, neck, head, and face. Which means, you can pretty much work on your entire body right now.

Do it for some time – however long you feel you need – with a relaxed and purposeful attitude.

Or you can stand up right now and practice for a bit.

Begin by imagining that you are standing here in uncharted territory without much knowledge of your body, much like a newborn baby who is learning how this body functions. You are marveling at its intricacy, and you are excited to explore it from head to toe. You are curious about everything. You are learning how to wiggle our toes and fingers. How exciting!

You are learning more and more about this body of yours that you were born into. You raise your arms and stretch higher and higher to reach for the magnificent stars and bend down lower and lower to reach for your glorious toes.

You rock back and forth, bend left and right, and learn how to keep your balance so you can remain standing upright. How joyful!

You breathe in and out, deeply, keeping the breath inside or outside for a while. You feel invigorated, blissful, full of life energy.

What better way of beginning your day can there possibly be? Except perhaps finding a winning Mega Lottery ticket on the sidewalk? Dream on.

During still, unmoving poses practice conscious muscle contractions. Do not move your joints or stretch your tendons. Us your conscious will and contract and relax the muscles while deeply breathing into and out of them.

Deep Belly Breathing

Perform deep belly breathing. Let your belly extend, relax all stomach muscles. Completely fill up with air, life, energy, fullness. Your stomach may resemble the extended belly of a very pregnant woman. Don't constrict your expansion. Put your palms on it and feel the muscles stretch on the slow deep inbreath.

Don't hold your breath after the inbreath or the outbreath. Just breathe in and out – ever deeper and deeper – like an inflating and deflating balloon.

If you get dizzy or light-headed, stop and resume your natural breath.

Follow The Breath

While placed in a basic position, follow the breath deep within, look around your body, and listen. Check on your joints, muscles, and tendons. See where they are at. This is like taking inventory, to see what you have to work with. Begin your exercise from this awareness of your body.

From here, work on any area that causes a problem, is a weakness, or a discomfort. See if you can work through it, or at least around it.

Avoid aggravating any discomfort or pain you feel. Seek to lesson those.

Above all, enjoy your time in this safe space of Extracise!

This is your sacred space, your most personal space. Everything you do here is totally YOU, every movement, every pose – moving or still, every breath, every muscle contraction and relaxation.

It is YOU, because this is your body, these are your joints, your muscles, your tendons, your breath, and your conscious will.

Thoughts On Holding Poses

When holding a position for a while, breathe deeply into it and shift your weight slightly from side to side, from front to back; always with a sense of balancing and centering your body.

Find the muscles that support you and keep you in balance. Breathe into them and contract them even more. Then relax those muscles to the point where they are just doing their job of balancing you safely.

Find the muscles that you don't need at the moment and contract and relax them consciously while breathing into and out of them. This will add to your workout, and it will increase your sense of wellbeing.

Compare left and right leaning movements, left and right twists. See if you can keep them even.

Before Bedtime

However tired you are, perform a few simple Extracises before going to bed. This will help you sleep better. Some simple stretches while breathing into them, some simple twists to loosen some strain from sitting too much. All done with gentle care.

And then, in bed, some easy muscle contractions while breathing into them. This will clear your head by taking your mind off other things.

Loading Of The Bones

Practice some loading of the bones. Standing in a doorway while pressing both arms up against the horizontal doorjamb. Press as hard as you can for a few seconds. Then slowly relax completely. This exercise helps with strengthening the bones of hands, arms, spine, hip, legs, and feet.

It is also a muscle strengthening exercise.

This Body

Our body is the vehicle that carries us through life.

Our bodies are designed for movement. The muscles act like little pumps that help with the blood flow through its arteries and veins. When you are sedentary, only your heart muscle drives the blood flow. That is why being sedentary is hard on your heart.

Any exercise can be enhanced by the principles of Extracise. Deep conscious breath. Full awareness of muscle contractions and relaxations. Full awareness of joint movements. Full engagement of your conscious will.

Flow of Chi

Every opportunity you have, stretch your spine, and make sure it is flexible. There are energy meridians located along the spine. A flexible spine ensures a smooth energy flow.

In order to feel the Chi flowing, put the palms and fingers of both hands together and breathe in and out of the connection between them.

Open palms mean your personal energy is flowing out into the universe. Closed palms mean your personal energy is contained within your body's energy system.

Human Efforts Towards Higher Aspiration

We humans have been given special qualities that give us the capacity to strive for higher achievements. Higher mentally, higher emotionally, higher spiritually. We are destined to always be seeking for the higher solution to any problem we encounter.

Our solutions must be higher, purer, with purer intentions, with the search for higher meanings, for everyone, for everything – including this entire planet and all of its inhabitants and lifeforms, however low on the evolutionary scale they may be, from simple microbes to grass to plants to all the insect and animal species, all the way to the spirits and gods.

Higher and higher. In everything we do, whether designing a wristwatch, tying our shoelaces, paying our taxes, authoring a novel, preaching a sermon, meditating, or breathing our final breath.

Always for the good of the one and the good of the many, and the good of the All. This is the universal principle – the cosmic principle – that is operating in this life that we are a part of. The never-ending strive for betterment on all levels; the achievement of greater-ness.

Sluggishness is the only enemy that we face, being lazy, uncommitted, letting minor and major things slide out of convenience and/or complacency.

Allowing for rot to set in, seeking our small selfish gains, trying to better other people so we can shine brighter, pulling others down so we appear greater.

Creating our own little world in which we are living a cocoon-like existence, cut off from the main strands of life. Searching only for our own happiness, grabbing our "share" of existence, and shutting the door to others once we walk through the gate into our garden of happiness. That is not what we should aspire to.

Primer On The Assemblage Point

This is a short introduction to a subject that has tremendous value to people attempting to improve their energetic profile.

The Assemblage Point is a concentrated energy field where all your personal energy experiences are concentrated. It is like the hub of a wheel, where all the spokes converge and where also all the spokes emanate.

This Assemblage Point can be considered your psychic energy center, where the conscious sense of self is located. It is located outside your body, but within its energy field, either to the left or the right side of your brain.

You can discover it when you carefully concentrate on it during quiet meditation. Sense and search around the area of your head and you will find it. You will get an energetic sensation of the place where it is.

This Assemblage Point can be moved to be in line with your chakras. That's where it should be, but because of habits and misinformation, it is not.

Use your hand and conscious will to move it to several inches above your head. Then use your pure intention to keep it there and become aware of how you feel. You may get a bit dizzy and disoriented from having your perspective of existence altered.

You may also feel and hear a slight cracking sound in your brain when you adjust the Point. This indicates an adjustment of your way of seeing the world.

To learn more about this interesting subject, go online and delve in.

Final Thoughts

My first encounter with a doctor was as a teenager. He told me that not every body part had to work perfectly. The important thing was that they all worked together in harmony, in balance. That is what constitutes physical health.

Always move towards inner glory, never towards outer glory. Examples of outer glory would be: the number of repetitions, the amount of weight lifted, the distance run, the trophies won, the height achieved, etc.

The movie "Chariots of Fire" is such a good example of inner glory versus outer glory. One of the athletes was striving for inner glory, the other for outer glory. The one striving for inner glory was consistently more content and at peace with himself than the other, outer driven athlete.

While practicing Extracise, please make certain you have a lot of fresh air. Keep a window open or practice outside in the open air.

You can add Extracise practices to your usual physical activities, like walking. You can lay down in bed before sleep or on a mat while sunbathing. Just add the conscious breath and your conscious will to tighten various muscles in your body.

I arrived at my system of Extracise by combining elements of Chi Kung, and Yoga. Both systems have still and moving forms. I added Isometrics to the mix to strengthen and invigorate individual muscles, and whole muscle groups.

Yoga is about making the body strong and flexible. Chi Kung is about directing vital energy into and through the body. Isometrics is about strengthening your muscles and your bones.

Breath is very important to me. The spine is very important to me. Stretching is very important to me. Reversal of bodily fluids is very important to me. Awareness is very important to me. Focus is very important to me.

Work around weaknesses and pains carefully, gently working through them. Weakness in muscles can lead to the body collapsing. Pain in a muscle can lead to a spasm, which is the muscle telling you it is going on strike and is now locking up.

Mobility of joints is important. Gently use your intention to create movement to loosen up the tendons to get maximum mobility. Don't force anything. If there is tension, gently work around it or through it. Make sure your muscles are warmed up. Don't ever force them to work while they are still cold.

Don't suppress burps and gas-letting. Often there is a gas built-up in your body, either in your stomach or your intestines. Gentle bends of your upper body can force these air bubbles out of your system. Don't feel embarrassed by that. One of the reasons why you practice Extracise is to cleanse your system of obstructions.

Consciously go through every part of your body and contract, stretch, and move your muscles, tendons, and joints.

Outer forms of exercises are guideposts indicating what your body is capable of doing. However, when you practice Extracise, you may go beyond these forms, or you may not get close to them. It all depends on the condition of your muscles, tendons, and joints. Don't push beyond your comfort level. You must remain in a state of concentrated ease, focused relaxation. Never under strain and tension.

Here is an advice and suggestion: don't ever focus on external achievements. Don't attempt to do a certain number of repetitions or get to a pre-determined distance. For example: don't do ten repetitions of something on a permanent basis. One day you may feel like nine repetitions, the next day like sixteen. Or you sign up for a marathon run. After mile eleven you decide you are losing your inner peace. So, you simply step aside and discontinue the race, call Uber and return home a happy person.

The ideal state produced by Extracise is when you are always in the relaxed state, your inner center, in your personal peaceful comfort zone. Yes, over time, you will extend this comfort zone, quite naturally, and you may decide to run longer than a marathon without giving it much thought, as long as you remain in your peaceful inner state.

This inner state is a state of calm-abiding and relaxed observing, while constantly adjusting to your present circumstances.

An important aspect of Extracise is complete relaxation of muscles and tendons. You start the Extracise from as close to a zero contraction or rotation as possible. Then you increase – slowly – gently, until you reach the max contraction or rotation.

Then you hold the position comfortably, perhaps coordinating it with your natural breath, and then you release the position comfortably until your muscles are back to being relaxed and your body is untwisted, back to where you started, to zero contraction and zero rotation. And then you can repeat. But always start from zero and end at zero. You do not want to start from an unknown state of contraction and end in an unknown state of relaxation. Your muscles need to be totally relaxed when you start and when you end your exercise.

You can practice large circular movement with your arms, hands, legs, torso, always with an emphasis on balance. Keep your eyes closed to increase your sense of balance.

Gentle rocking motions while holding a pose is beneficial in gently stretching muscles and tendons.

Combine this with natural breathing. It is very calming, very soothing.

Always stay in your own rhythm. Find it, find your speed, your effort, which is uniquely yours. Don't overstep your rhythm. Remain in it. Don't follow someone else's rhythm. Find your own rhythm in everything you do, think, feel, act, project, originate, create. Your life – your rhythm.

Get into your own zone! Remain in it even if you are facing ridicule, or criticism, or pressure, or opposition. Remain firm in your rhythm, but also flexible to allow for change – and change always comes, new thoughts come, new world views come, new realizations dawn.

Release muscle tensions slowly, not abruptly. Your blood pressure could drop too fast if you release contracted muscles too quickly, resulting in dizziness and diminished physical coordination.

Problems with imbalance in your body activities can take years to develop into symptoms of discomfort and pain. Or you can feel them immediately and are able to correct them appropriately.

But with the long-term imbalances, the causes of your present pain are often not easily diagnosed. Keeping a journal may help you to see when the first slight sensation of the discomfort arose.

And ... The Wrap-up

The mission, so to speak, of Extracise is fourfold:

1. Consciously move or rotate every joint.

2. Consciously contract and relax every muscle.

3. Consciously stretch every muscle and tendon.

4. Consciously use the breath to energize your entire body.

5. Utilize the conscious will almost exclusively to practice. Do not fall into a mindless routine without the clearest awareness of your practices.

Yoga is defined as "Stilling of the thought-ripples of the mind." So, when you practice your Extracises, keep that in mind. Stop worrying. Stop thinking and get into the state of being. Experience the exercises fully!

Other Books By The Author

Handbook of Consciousness – Vijnana Bhairava Meditations

LISTENING – The Art of Self-Inquiry

There is Only One

Liberation – A few Words to the Wise

The Moment of Perfection

Contact Information

If you want to contact me, send an email to:

Extracise123@gmail.com

www.ingramcontent.com/pod-product-compliance
Lightning Source LLC
Chambersburg PA
CBHW070848250726

48662CB00003B/1422